Couch to Fit

Two Month Beginner Gym Program

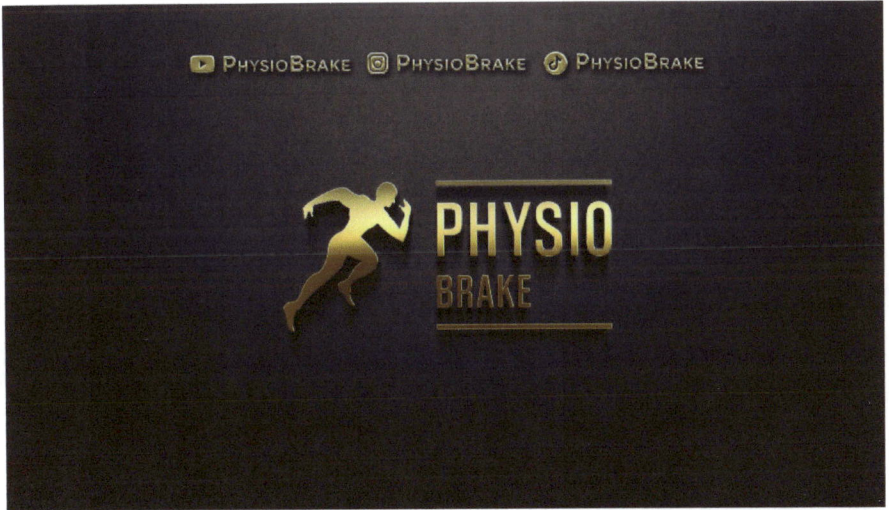

ABOUT THE AUTHOR

I am a Registered Physical Therapist with a passion for advancing the accessibility of fitness for everyone. This gym-based program is for any individual looking to step foot into the gym for the first time or someone who has been in the gym before, but never had their own program. This program focuses on key muscle groups for injury prevention, muscle strength, and overall fitness.

Christopher Brake MPT BSc
Registered Physical Therapist

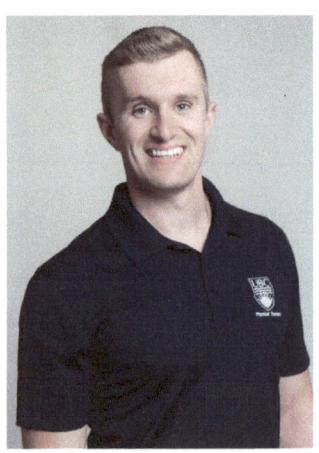

Embracing Fitness

Getting started, going from the couch to the gym, is the hardest step in your fitness journey. In our busy lives, it's easy for health goals to get pushed aside. But finding the right balance between life's demands and a solid workout routine is key to staying energized and ready for whatever challenges may come your way. It is important for increasing your life battery and improving your resilience when participating in the activities you enjoy. Join me, as we take the plunge to starting your fitness journey together.

Making Time for Rest and Relaxation

As we know, life is a whirlwind of activities and responsibilities, but it's crucial to remember the importance of rest, recovery, and relaxation. Just as your body needs breaks between workouts to get stronger, your mind also needs moments of calm and self-care to stay refreshed.

The Benefits of Exercise

Exercise, especially weight training, isn't just about looking good—it's about feeling great and staying healthy. It provides a dependable routine and a sense of accomplishment amidst daily challenges. Weightlifting boosts your metabolism, strengthens your bones, and enhances overall endurance. These benefits go beyond the gym, improving your posture, reducing injury risks, and boosting your confidence in everyday life.

Resistance Exercise:
- **Improves Physical Health**: Strengthens the heart, lungs, and muscles, reducing the risk of chronic diseases.
- **Boosts Mental Health**: Reduces symptoms of anxiety and depression, enhancing mood and overall mental well-being.
- **Aids Weight Management**: Helps maintain a healthy weight by burning calories and increasing metabolism.
- **Increases Energy Levels**: Boosts stamina and reduces fatigue, making daily activities easier.
- **Enhances Sleep Quality**: Promotes better sleep patterns, helping you fall asleep faster and sleep more deeply.
- **Strengthens Bones and Muscles**: Improves bone density and muscle strength, reducing the risk of osteoporosis.
- **Improves Brain Function**: Enhances cognitive function and memory and may reduce the risk of cognitive decline.
- **Promotes Social Connections**: Provides opportunities to meet new people through group activities or classes.
- **Boosts Immune Function**: Regular exercise can strengthen the immune system, helping to ward off illnesses.
- **Increases Longevity**: Linked to a longer lifespan and a higher quality of life as you age.

Skeletal Muscle

A basic understanding of muscle function is important to optimize any exercise routine.

Skeletal muscle is characterized by its striated appearance and is composed of long, cylindrical fibers. Skeletal muscles crave movement and load and will adapt to many of the stresses put on to them. Fortunately, skeletal muscle is under voluntary control, meaning movements can be consciously initiated. This includes walking, lifting, and running. Skeletal muscles work in pairs, known as antagonistic pairs, where one muscle contracts while the other relaxes, enabling coordinated movement at joints.

The organization of skeletal muscle into bundles, called fascicles, is surrounded by connective tissues that provide support and protection. Each muscle fiber contains myofibrils, which consist of repeating units called sarcomeres, the fundamental units of contraction. These sarcomeres contain the proteins actin (thin filaments) and myosin (thick filaments) that interact during contraction through the sliding filament theory.

Muscle Organization and Function

The entire muscle is encased in a tougher layer known as the epimysium. Tendons, which are made of dense connective tissue, attach muscles to bones, enabling the transfer of force when muscles contract. This connection is crucial for producing movement at joints, where skeletal muscles play a primary role. Just like muscles, tendons also adapt to load and appropriate stress.

Muscles are highly vascularized to meet their energy demands, with an extensive network of blood vessels supplying oxygen and nutrients. During physical activity, increased blood flow to muscles supports the heightened metabolic activity required for sustained contractions. Each skeletal muscle fiber is innervated by a motor neuron at a specialized junction known as the neuromuscular junction, where the release of neurotransmitters initiates contraction.

Key Functions of Muscles

The primary functions of muscles include movement and stability. Muscles enable voluntary and involuntary movements essential for daily activities and complex actions. They also contribute to maintaining posture and stabilizing joints, preventing injuries during movement.

In summary, muscle anatomy is a complex and essential aspect of human biology, with each type of muscle tissue fulfilling specific roles. Together, they support movement, stability, and vital bodily functions, underscoring the importance of muscles in maintaining overall health and performance.

The length of time it takes to see muscle benefits from exercise can vary based on several factors, including the type of exercise, frequency, intensity, individual fitness levels, nutrition, and recovery.

Staying on Track Without Losing Momentum

Navigating life's busy seasons doesn't mean abandoning our fitness aspirations. Instead, it invites us to adopt a balanced approach that honors both our physical goals and the demands of everyday life. Whether it's carving out time for a brisk walk or enjoying a peaceful yoga session, integrating exercise into our routine can be both invigorating and uplifting.

Couch to Fit: YouTube Demonstrations
This QR-code will bring you to my YouTube channel where I talk through the program in more detail, provide demonstrations and clear explanations of key terms and themes.

A Healthier, Happier You

As we embrace the gift of fitness, let's remember that staying active isn't just about maintaining a certain physique—it's about nurturing our well-being and enjoying the benefits of movement. By finding harmony between indulgence and discipline, we can enjoy life's pleasures without guilt while laying the foundation for a healthier, happier future.

So, here's to celebrating with vigor, embracing our inner strength, and ensuring that our journey through this period leaves us not only motivated but also on track to achieve our fitness goals. Let's toast to health, happiness, and the gains we make along the way!

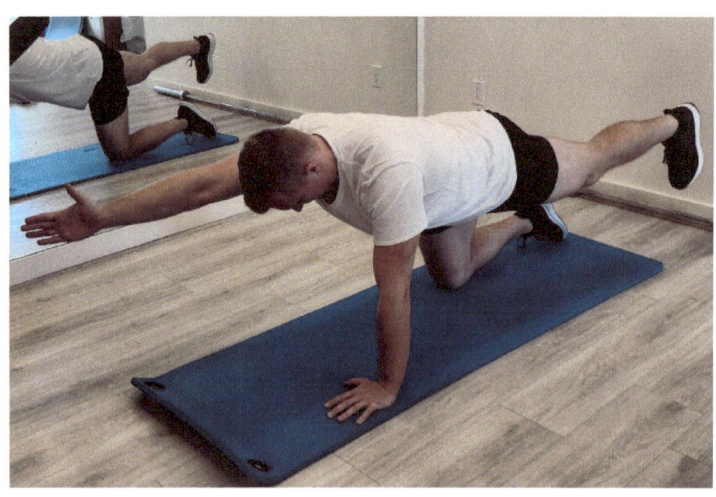

Table of Contents

How To Use This Program	10
Key Terms	10
Week One	15
Week Two	18
Week Three	21
Week Four	24
Week Five	27
Week Six	30
Week Seven	33
Week Eight	36
Exercise Tracking Sheet	38
Mobility & Stretching Routine	40
Conclusion	41
Exercise Descriptions	42

How to Use this Program:

I designed this program for people unfamiliar with the gym and don't know where to start. But even if you know your way around, this program gives you safe, progressive training from a Physical Therapist's point of view.

The idea of this program is to help build confidence in the gym setting and learn the basic movements and machines to develop a great exercise foundation.

The exercises chosen are injury preventative and help to build muscular strength, endurance and improve overall fitness.

Each week will have coaching tips provided to help guide how it should feel during that week, things to focus on and what is to be expected.

Start: Muscle Adaptation

This program is 8 weeks long. The initial 4 weeks consist of maximizing the connections between body and brain (neurological improvements). With the first 2 weeks focus on more endurance and technique of the exercises (lower sets and higher reps). The last 4 weeks will be adaptation to the muscles (improved muscle size, endurance, strength). This is a normal adaptation timeline for any person beginning any program.

As the weeks progress from Week 1 to 8, the exercises shift to more strength and hypertrophy. Keep an eye on which week you are on and the required reps for each exercise on the table.

Additionally, there are three days that are recommended for focusing on cardiovascular health, muscle mobility and flexibility. This should **NOT** be skipped. As good cardiovascular health improves blood flow and nutrients to the muscles for growth and recovery.

2 for 2 Rule: Progressive Overload

It is very important to always use an appropriate amount of weight for each exercise. When choosing a weight or resistance, the weight should feel challenging on the last two reps, but you are still able to successfully complete the set. If you perform the same weight on an exercise for two consecutive days and the last two reps are no longer challenging, then it is time to increase the resistance. So, the last two reps of the set are always challenging. This is the theory of progressive overload.
- Increase upper body resistance by no more than 5lbs.
- Increase lower body resistance by no more than 10lbs.

Gym Days:

Before every workout you will be encouraged to do a warm-up routine (**see the end of the book**) and after each workout a light stretch and cool down (**see the end of this book**). The gym days are weight-training based, with recovery days focused on cardiovascular health.

Key Terms: Used in the Exercise Day Tables Below

DB: Dumbbell – Single hand weights

BB: Barbell – Long two-handed bar

KB: Kettlebell – Bell shaped weight with handle on top

CB: Cable – Pulley system or can be resistance bands

MC: Machine – Various gym machines and equipment that are set up for specific exercise

AMRAP: As many reps as possible

TIME: Holding for as long as possible

Exercise: The movement you are to perform

Repetitions: The number of times you will repeat the exercise at once

Sets: The number of groupings you will perform of that exercise

Rest: Time between each set of exercises

Weight: Tracking the amount of weight used for each exercise (See above 2 for 2 Rule)

*: This will denote any changes to an exercise from the previous week.

Week One: Coaching Tips

Remember, this is your first week. The emphasis is on starting small and building up slowly. I want you to prioritize starting with two sets per exercise.

The 15 reps are the goal, but if you can do 12, 10 or just 8, that is also excellent. Starting small and then building up repetitions is **KEY**.

Since this is a new program for you, expect some muscle soreness the day after exercises. This is called delayed onset muscle soreness, and it is totally normal.

Most gyms will have images on the machines (MC), for the MC exercises, such as the MC Chest press. Please ask gym attendants to help as I did not take videos or photos of the MC exercises.

The end of the document shows pictures for some of the niche exercises not linked by the QR code in my YouTube Demonstrations.

Week One
Gym Days (See end for Warm-up & Cool-Down)
Day One: Chest, Triceps, Core

Exercise	Sets	Reps	Rest	Weight
MC Chest Press	3	15	1 min	Light
MC Chest Fly	2	15	1 min	Light
Push-Ups	3	AMRAP	1 min	Body
DB Incline Press	2	15	1 min	Light
CB Press downs	2	15	1 min	Light
High Plank	2	TIME	30 seconds	Body

Day Two: Legs & Core

Exercise	Sets	Reps	Rest	Weight
DB Squat	3	15	1 min	Light
KB Deadlift	2	15	1 min	Light
Reverse Lunge	2	15	1 min	Body
Side Lunge	2	15	1 min	Body
Heel Raises off Step	2	20	1 min	Body
Glute Bridge	2	16	1 min	Body
Dead bug	2	16	30 seconds	Body

Day Three: Back, Biceps, Shoulders

Exercise	Sets	Reps	Rest	Weight
MC Back Row	3	15	1 min	Light
CB Lat Pulldown	2	15	1 min	Light
DB Shoulder Press	2	15	1 min	Light
DB Lateral Raise	2	15	1 min	Light
DB Shoulder Rotation	2	15	1 min	Light
DB Curl	2	15	1 min	Light

Day Four Back, Shoulders & Legs

Exercise	Sets	Reps	Rest	Weight
MC Quad Ext	3	15	1 min	Light
MC Hamstring	3	15	1 min	Light
Hip Abduction	3	15	1 min	Light
CB Row	3	15	1 min	Light
CB Shoulder Lateral Rotation	2	15	1 min	Light
CB Shoulder Medial Rotation	2	15	1 min	Light

Week One: Recovery Days (Gym Rest Days)

Day One:
- ☐ Walk or Run for Total of 10 minutes (2 times of 5 minutes or 1 burst of 10)
- ☐ Mobility Routine Upper and Lower body (**See end of Document**)

Day Two:
- ☐ Either walk or run for a total of 10 minutes, or
- ☐ Try a stationary bike or elliptical at the gym
- ☐ Stretching Routine Upper and Lower Body (**See end of Document**)

Day Three:
- ☐ Do something fun! Have a good warm-up, try a new sport, do a little hike, go for a swim or something new
- ☐ Mobility and/or Stretching
- ☐ Challenge yourself with a longer walk!

Week Two: Coaching Tips

For this week we are trying to build our reps up to be closer to 15 per set. If you did 8 reps last week, try 10 reps. If you did 10, try 12. And so on. We are still focusing on good form and using lighter weight to build our foundation.

Building muscular endurance is our first goal. Remember the **2 for 2 rule** I described for progression overload in the beginning. It is critical to safely progress reps and weight. Watch the video link in the QR code for a clearer explanation of progressive overload.

You should still expect to feel muscle soreness the day after exercises, but it should dissipate within 24 hours – 48 hours.

Drink water, eat well, sleep lots.

Week Two
Day One: Chest, Triceps, Core

Exercise	Sets	Reps	Rest	Weight
MC Chest Press	3	15	1 min	Light
MC Chest Fly	2	15	1 min	Light
Push-Ups	3	AMRAP	1 min	Body
DB Incline Press	2	15	1 min	Light
CB Press downs	2	15	1 min	Light
High Plank	2	TIME	30 seconds	Body

Day Two: Legs & Core

Exercise	Sets	Reps	Rest	Weight
DB Squat	3	15	1 min	Light
KB Deadlift	2	15	1 min	Light
Reverse Lunge	2	15	1 min	Body
Side Lunge	2	15	1 min	Body
Heel Raises off Step	2	20	1 min	Body
Glute Bridge	2	16	1 min	Body
Dead bug	2	16	30 seconds	Body

Day Three: Back, Biceps, Shoulders

Exercise	Sets	Reps	Rest	Weight
MC Back Row	3	15	1 min	Light
CB Lat Pulldown	2	15	1 min	Light
DB Shoulder Press	2	15	1 min	Light
DB Lateral Raise	2	15	1 min	Light
DB Shoulder Rotation	2	15	1 min	Light
DB Curl	2	15	1 min	Light

Day Four: Back, Shoulders & Legs

Exercise	Sets	Reps	Rest	Weight
MC Quad Ext	3	15	1 min	Light
MC Hamstring	3	15	1 min	Light
MC Hip Abduction	3	15	1 min	Light
CB Row	3	15	1 min	Light
CB Shoulder Lateral Rotation	2	15	1 min	Light
CB Shoulder Medial Rotation	2	15	1 min	Light
CB Shoulder Lateral Rotation	2	15	1 min	Light

Week Two: Recovery Days (Gym Rest Days)
Day One:

- Walk or Run for Total of 15 minutes (2 - 3 times of 5 minutes or 1 burst of 10 - 15)
- Mobility Routine Upper and Lower body (**See end of Document**)

Day Two:

- Either walk or run for a total of 15 minutes, or
- Try a stationary bike or elliptical at the gym
- Stretching Routine Upper and Lower Body (**See end of Document**)

Day Three:

- Do something fun! Have a good warm-up, try a new sport, do a little hike, go for a swim or something new
- You can always try a bigger walk!
- Mobility and/or Stretching

Week Three: Coaching Tips

Now we should be at the 15 reps. Possibly even performing a third set for some of the exercises.

The workout should start to feel a little easier. Our nervous system is adapting to the exercises between weeks 1 – 4. So, these initial strength and rep gains we are feeling are due to our brain better utilizing the muscle we already have.

It is critical to have proper rest and nutrition. The program is designed to have rest days in-between. This helps muscle recovery. Try your best to find a good balance in your schedule.

It takes three weeks to build a habit. Solidify this third week into your routine.

Week Three
Day One: Chest, Triceps, Core

Exercise	Sets	Reps	Rest	Weight
DB* Chest Press	3	15	1 min	Light
MC Chest Fly	3	15	1 min	Light
Push-Ups	3	AMRAP	1 min	Body
DB Incline Press	3	15	1 min	Light
CB Press downs	3	15	1 min	Light
Low Plank*	3	TIME	30 seconds	Body
Side Plank*	2	TIME	30 seconds	Body

Day Two: Legs & Core

Exercise	Sets	Reps	Rest	Weight
DB Squat	3	15	1 min	Light
KB Deadlift	3	15	1 min	Light
DB Reverse Lunge	3	15	1 min	Light
KB* Side Lunge	3	15	1 min	Light
DB* Heel Raises off Step	3	20	1 min	Light
Glute Bridge	3	16	1 min	Body
Dead bug	3	16	30 secs	Body

Day Three: Back, Biceps, Shoulders

Exercise	Sets	Reps	Rest	Weight
MC Back Row	3	15	1 min	Light
CB Lat Pull Down	3	15	1 min	Light
DB Bent Over Row	3	15	1 min	Light
DB Shoulder Press	3	15	1 min	Light
DB Lateral Raise	3	15	1 min	Light
DB Front Raise	3	15	1 min	Light
DB Curl	3	15	1 min	Light

Day Four: Back, Shoulders & Legs

Exercise	Sets	Reps	Rest	Weight
Leg Press*	3	15	1 min	Light
MC Hamstring	3	15	1 min	Light
Hip Abduction	3	15	1 min	Light
CB Seated Row	3	15	1 min	Light
CB Shoulder Lateral Rotation	3	15	1 min	Light
CB Shoulder Medial Rotation	3	15	1 min	Light
MC Reverse Fly	3	15	1 min	Light

Week Three: Recovery Days (Gym Rest Days)
Day One:
- Walk or Run for Total of 20 minutes (2 times of 10 minutes or 1 burst of 20)
- Mobility Routine Upper and Lower body (**See end of Document**)

Day Two:
- Either walk or run for a total of 20 minutes, or
- Try a stationary bike or elliptical at the gym
- Stretching Routine Upper and Lower Body (**See end of Document**)

Day Three:
- Do something fun! Have a good warm-up, try a new sport, do a little hike, go for a swim or something new
- You can always try a bigger walk!

Week Four: Coaching Tips

We are nearing the halfway mark, and this is the first week I want you to start using a **MODERATE (Mod)** amount of weight. This should be heavy enough that 10 to 12 reps feel like a challenge (as described in my introduction and intro videos).

Example: If you DB Chest pressed 20lbs week 3 for 15 reps, it would be fair to say that is too easy for 10 – 12 rep targets. If you increase your weight to 30lbs and can only get 6 reps, then that is too heavy. Find the weight that you can successfully do 10 to 12 reps with a challenge on the last two reps.

The key for this week is to adjust the reps and weight to be challenging for the 10 to 12 rep range. We are now working on muscle **hypertrophy and strength**, stepping away from endurance. Muscle DOMS are expected to post workouts now.

For increasing weight, I like to increase the upper body by no more than 5lbs a session and lower body by 5 – 10 lbs a session.

Week Four
Day One: Chest, Triceps, Core

Exercise	Sets	Reps	Rest	Weight
DB Chest Press	3	10 - 12	1 min	Mod
MC Chest Fly	3	10 - 12	1 min	Mod
Push-Ups	3	AMRAP	1 min	Body
DB Incline Press	3	10 - 12	1 min	Mod
CB Press downs	3	10 - 12	1 min	Mod
Low Plank	3	TIME	30 seconds	Body
Side Plank	2	TIME	30 seconds	Body

Day Two: Legs & Core

Exercise	Sets	Reps	Rest	Weight
DB Squat	3	10 - 12	1 min	Mod
KB Deadlift	3	10 - 12	1 min	Mod
DB Reverse Lunge	3	10 - 12	1 min	Mod
KB Side Lunge	3	10 - 12	1 min	Mod
DB Heel Raises off Step	3	16	1 min	Mod
Glute Bridge	3	16	1 min	Body
Dead bug	3	20	30 sec	Body

Day Three: Back, Biceps, Shoulders

Exercise	Sets	Reps	Rest	Weight
MC Back Row	3	10 - 12	1 min	Mod
CB Lat Pulldown	3	10 - 12	1 min	Mod
DB Bent Over Row	3	10 - 12	1 min	Mod
DB Shoulder Press	3	10 - 12	1 min	Mod
DB Lateral Raise	3	10 - 12	1 min	Mod
DB Front Raise	3	10 - 12	1 min	Mod
DB Curl	3	10 - 12	1 min	Mod

Day Four: Back, Shoulders & Legs

Exercise	Sets	Reps	Rest	Weight
Leg Press	3	10 - 12	1 min	Mod
MC Hamstring	3	10 - 12	1 min	Mod
Hip Abduction	3	10 - 12	1 min	Mod
CB Seated Row	3	10 - 12	1 min	Mod
CB Shoulder Lateral Rotation	3	10 - 12	1 min	Mod
CB Shoulder Medial Rotation	3	10 - 12	1 min	Mod
MC Reverse Fly	3	10 - 12	1 min	Mod

Week Four: Recovery Days (Gym Rest Days)
Day One:
- Walk or Run for Total of 30 minutes (2 times of 15 minutes or 1 burst of 30)
- Mobility Routine Upper and Lower body (**See end of Document**)

Day Two:
- Either walk or run for a total of 30 minutes, or
- Try a stationary bike or elliptical at the gym
- Stretching Routine Upper and Lower Body (**See end of Document**)

Day Three:
- Do something fun! Have a good warm-up, try a new sport, do a little hike, go for a swim or something new!
- You can always try a bigger walk!
- Mobility and/or Stretching (**See end of Document**)

Week Five: Coaching Tips

Most exercise sets should be at 3 sets now. You should be noticing you are getting stronger and using heavier weights than when your started out.

It is critical that you adjust the weight accordingly to hit the 10 – 12 rep range. You may need to increase your weight more than you think to feel appropriate fatigue for the 10 to 12 reps.

For increasing weight, I like to increase the upper body by no more than 5lbs a session and lower body by 5 – 10 lbs a session.

At this stage of working out, some people may find increased fatigue. It is natural that after 4 to 6 weeks of consistent weight training to have a natural dip in energy. This is a good time to reflect on your rest and recovery, your sleep and nutrition. If an extra rest day is required to be successful, then please don't hesitate to take it.

Week Five
Day One: Chest, Triceps, Core

Exercise	Sets*	Reps	Rest	Weight*
DB Chest Press	3	10 - 12	1 min	Mod
MC Chest Fly	3	10 - 12	1 min	Mod
Push-Ups	3	AMRAP	1 min	Body
DB Incline Press	3	10 - 12	1 min	Mod
CB Press downs	3	10 - 12	1 min	Mod
Low Plank	3	TIME	30 sec	Body
Side Plank	2	TIME	30 sec	Body

Day Two: Legs & Core

Exercise	Sets	Reps	Rest	Weight
DB Squat	3	10 - 12	1 min	Mod
KB Deadlift	3	10 - 12	1 min	Mod
DB Reverse Lunge	3	10 - 12	1 min	Mod
KB Side Lunge	3	10 - 12	1 min	Mod
Single Leg Heel Raise*	3	16	1 min	Mod
Band Glute Bridge	3	16	1 min	Body
Dead bug	3	20	30sec	Body

Day Three: Back, Biceps, Shoulders

Exercise	Sets	Reps	Rest	Weight
MC Back Row	3	10 - 12	1 min	Mod
CB Lat Pulldown	3	10 - 12	1 min	Mod
DB Bent Over Row	3	10 - 12	1 min	Mod
DB Shoulder Press	3	10 - 12	1 min	Mod
DB Lateral Raise	3	10 - 12	1 min	Mod
DB Front Raise	3	10 - 12	1 min	Mod
DB Curl	3	10 - 12	1 min	Mod

Day Four: Back, Shoulders & Legs

Exercise	Sets	Reps	Rest	Weight
Leg Press	3	10 - 12	1 min	Mod
MC Hamstring	3	10 - 12	1 min	Mod
Hip Abduction	3	10 - 12	1 min	Mod
CB Seated Row	3	10 - 12	1 min	Mod
CB Shoulder Lateral Rotation	3	10 - 12	1 min	Mod
CB Shoulder Medial Rotation	3	10 - 12	1 min	Mod
MC Reverse Fly	3	10 - 12	1 min	Mod

Week Five: Recovery Days (Gym Rest Days)
Day One:
- Walk or Run for Total of 30 - 35 minutes (2 times of 15 - 20 minutes or 1 burst of 35)
- Mobility Routine Upper and Lower body (**See end of Document**)

Day Two:
- Either walk or run for a total of 30 - 35 minutes, or
- Try a stationary bike or elliptical at the gym
- Stretching Routine Upper and Lower Body (**See end of Document**)

Day Three:
- Do something fun! Have a good warm-up, try a new sport, do a little hike, go for a swim or something new
- You can always try a bigger walk!
- Mobility and/or Stretching

Week Six: Coaching Tips

Big changes this week as we again **increase the weight** to be between moderate and heavy. Now we are focusing on the reps being between 8 to 12 reps.

Try picking a weight that makes it so 8 reps is challenging. Again, remember the 2 for 2 rule that was described in the beginning of this document.

Build those 8 reps up to 12 reps, then increase the weight and repeat the cycle from 8 reps.

Example: DB Squat 3 sets x 8 reps of 40lbs.
The next week I will go up to 10 reps, and then 12 reps at 40lbs. Once I am at 3 sets x 12 reps x 40lbs, I will then increase the weight to 45lbs but reduce my reps back to 8. Then repeat the cycling building back up to 12 reps.

Week Six
Day One: Chest, Triceps, Core

Exercise	Sets	Reps	Rest	Weight
DB Chest Press	3	8 - 12	1 min 30	Mod
MC Chest Fly	3	8 - 12	1 min 30	Mod
Push-Ups	3	AMRAP	1 min	Body
DB Incline Press	3	8 - 12	1 min 30	Mod
CB Press downs	3	8 - 12	1 min	Mod
Low Plank	3	TIME	30 seconds	Body
Side Plank	2	TIME	30 seconds	Body

Day Two: Legs & Core

Exercise	Set	Reps	Rest	Weight
DB Squat	3	8 - 12	90 sec	Mod
KB Deadlift	3	8 - 12	90 sec	Mod
DB Reverse Lunge	3	8 - 12	90 sec	Mod
KB Side Lunge	3	8 - 12	90 sec	Mod
Single Leg Heel Raise	3	15	1 min	Mod
Band Glute Bridge	3	16	1 min	Body
Dead bug	3	20	30 sec	Body

Day Three: Back, Biceps, Shoulders

Exercise	Sets	Reps	Rest	Weight
MC Back Row	3	8 - 12	1 min 30	Mod
CB Lat Pulldown	3	8 - 12	1 min 30	Mod
DB Bent Over Row	3	8 - 12	1 min 30	Mod
DB Shoulder Press	3	8 - 12	1 min 30	Mod
DB Lateral Raise	3	8 - 12	1 min	Mod
DB Front Raise	3	8 - 12	1 min	Mod
DB Curl	3	8 - 12	1 min	Mod

Day Four: Back, Shoulders & Legs

Exercise	Sets	Reps	Rest	Weight*
Leg Press	3	8 - 12	90 secs	Mod to Heavy
MC Hamstring	3	8 - 12	1 min	Mod to Heavy
Hip Abduction	3	8 - 12	1 min	Mod to Heavy
CB Seated Row	3	8 - 12	90 secs	Mod to Heavy
CB Shoulder Lateral Rotation	3	8 - 12	1 min	Mod to Heavy
CB Shoulder Medial Rotation	3	8 - 12	1 min	Mod to Heavy
MC Reverse Fly	3	8 - 12	1 min	Mod to Heavy

Week Six: Recovery Days (Gym Rest Days)
Day One:
- Walk or Run for Total of 35 minutes (2 times of 15 - 20 minutes or 1 burst of 35)
- Mobility Routine Upper and Lower body (**See end of Document**)

Day Two:
- Either walk or run for a total of 35 minutes, or
- Try a stationary bike or elliptical at the gym
- Stretching Routine Upper and Lower Body (**See end of Document**)

Day Three:
- Do something fun! Have a good warm-up, try a new sport, do a little hike, go for a swim or something new
- You can always try a bigger walk!
- Mobility and/or Stretching

Week Seven: Coaching Tips

If you have made it to week seven, congratulations, you are making long term adaptations. I am proud of you. You are truly doing this thing.

Continue with the concepts from week six, trying to keep the weights challenging for the 8 to 12 reps.

At this stage, you and others may start to notice changes happening in your body as muscles are building.

Week Seven
Day One: Chest, Triceps, Core

Exercise	Sets	Reps	Rest	Weight*
DB Chest Press	3	8 - 12	1 min 30	Mod
MC Chest Fly	3	8 - 12	1 min 30	Mod
Push-Ups	3	AMRAP	1 min	Body
DB Incline Press	3	8 - 12	1 min	Mod
CB Press downs	3	8 - 12	1 min	Mod
Low Plank	3	TIME	30	Body
Side Plank	2	TIME	30	Body

Day Two: Legs & Core

Exercise	Sets	Reps	Rest	Weight*
DB Squat	3	8 - 12	1 min 30	Mod
KB Deadlift	3	8 - 12	1 min 30	Mod
DB Reverse Lunge	3	8 - 12	1 min 30	Mod
KB Side Lunge	3	8 - 12	1 min	Mod
Single Leg Heel Raise	3	15	1 min	Mod
Band Glute Bridge	3	16	1 min	Body
Dead bug	3	20	30 sec	Body

Day Three: Back, Biceps, Shoulders

Exercise	Sets	Reps	Rest	Weight*
MC Back Row	3	8 - 12	1 min 30	Mod
CB Lat Pulldown	3	8 - 12	1 min 30	Mod
DB Bent Over Row	3	8 - 12	1 min 30	Mod
DB Shoulder Press	3	8 - 12	1 min 30	Mod
DB Lateral Raise	3	8 - 12	1 min	Mod
DB Front Raise	3	8 - 12	1 min	Mod
DB Curl	3	8 - 12	1 min	Mod

Day Four: Back, Shoulders & Legs

Exercise	Sets	Reps	Rest	Weight*
Leg Press	3	8 - 12	90 secs	Mod to Heavy
MC Hamstring	3	8 - 12	1 min	Mod to Heavy
Hip Abduction	3	8 - 12	1 min	Mod to Heavy
CB Seated Row	3	8 - 12	90 secs	Mod to Heavy
CB Shoulder Lateral Rotation	3	8 - 12	1 min	Mod to Heavy
CB Shoulder Medial Rotation	3	8 - 12	1 min	Mod to Heavy
MC Reverse Fly	3	8 - 12	1 min	Mod to Heavy

Week Seven: Recovery Days (Gym Rest Days)

Day One:
- Walk or Run for Total of 35 minutes (2 times of 15 - 20 minutes or 1 burst of 35)
- Mobility Routine Upper and Lower body (**See end of Document**)

Day Two:
- Either walk or run for a total of 35 minutes, or
- Try a stationary bike or elliptical at the gym
- Stretching Routine Upper and Lower Body (**See end of Document**)

Day Three:
- Do something fun! Have a good warm-up, try a new sport, do a little hike, go for a swim or something new
- You can always try a bigger walk!
- Mobility and/or Stretching

Week Eight: Coaching Tips

We are on the last week! Finish strong!

This is where things get interesting...

You should now notice changes in your body, more strength, change of body fat composition and overall better health. You cannot stop here. This is just the beginning. What you can do is continue to do week 8 for as long as you need to, progressing the weights until you find my next program: Fit to Barbell Basics!

We have built that habit over the last 8 weeks and we need to make this a life-style thing!

Week Eight
Day One: Chest, Triceps, Core

Exercise	Sets	Reps	Rest	Weight
DB Bench Press	3	8 - 12	2 mins	Mod
DB Chest Fly*	3	8 - 12	1 min 30	Mod
Push-Ups	3	AMRAP	1 min	Body
DB Incline Press	3	8 - 12	1 min	Mod
CB Press downs	3	8 - 12	1 min	Mod
Low Plank	3	TIME	30 sec	Body
Side Plank	2	TIME	30 sec	Body

Day Two: Legs & Core

Exercise	Sets	Reps	Rest	Weight
DB Squat	3	8 - 12	2 mins	Mod
KB Deadlift	3	8 - 12	1 min	Mod
DB Reverse Lunge	3	8 - 12	1 min	Mod
KB Side Lunge	3	8 - 12	1 min	Mod
Single Leg Heel Raise	3	15	1 min	Mod
Band Glute Bridge	3	16	1 min	Body
Dead bug	3	20	30 sec	Body

Day Three: Back, Biceps, Shoulders

Exercise	Sets	Reps	Rest	Weight
BB Back Row	3	8 - 12	2 mins	Mod
CB Lat Pulldown	3	8 - 12	1 min 30	Mod
DB Bent Over Row	3	8 - 12	1 min 30	Mod
DB Shoulder Press	3	8 - 12	1 min 30	Mod
DB Lateral Raise	3	8 - 12	1 min	Mod
DB Front Raise	3	8 - 12	1 min	Mod
DB Curl	3	8 - 12	1 min	Mod

Day Four: Back, Shoulders & Legs

Exercise	Sets	Reps	Rest	Weight*
Leg Press	3	8 - 12	90 secs	Mod to Heavy
MC Hamstring	3	8 - 12	1 min	Mod to Heavy
Hip Abduction	3	8 - 12	1 min	Mod to Heavy
CB Seated Row	3	8 - 12	90 secs	Mod to Heavy
CB Shoulder Lateral Rotation	3	8 - 12	1 min	Mod to Heavy
CB Shoulder Medial Rotation	3	8 - 12	1 min	Mod to Heavy
MC Reverse Fly	3	8 - 12	1 min	Mod to Heavy

Week Eight: Recovery Days (Gym Rest Days)
Day One:
- Walk or Run for Total of 35 - 45 minutes (2 times of 20 minutes or 1 burst of 35 - 45)
- Mobility Routine Upper and Lower body (**See end of Document**)

Day Two:
- Either walk or run for a total of 35 minutes, or
- Try a stationary bike or elliptical at the gym
- Stretching Routine Upper and Lower Body (**See end of Document**)

Day Three:
- Do something fun! Have a good warm-up, try a new sport, do a little hike, go for a swim or something new
- You can always try a bigger walk!
- Mobility and/or Stretching

Exercise Tracking Sheet – Weeks 1-4

Week	Day	Date	Exercise 1	Exercise 2	Exercise 3	Exercise 4	Exercise 5	Exercise 6
1	1							
1	2							
1	3							
2	1							
2	2							
2	3							
3	1							
3	2							
3	3							
4	1							
4	2							
4	3							

Exercise Tracking Sheet – Weeks 5-8

Week	Day	Date	Exercise 1	Exercise 2	Exercise 3	Exercise 4	Exercise 5	Exercise 6
5	1							
5	2							
5	3							
6	1							
6	2							
6	3							
7	1							
7	2							
7	3							
8	1							
8	2							
8	3							

Mobility & Stretching Routine

Mobility is recommended to be done before the gym and other activities to help warm-up the joint throughout a full range of motion.

Stretching is recommended to be completed after activities to help the muscles cool down and aids in muscle recovery.

Mobility Routine: Upper Body

Arm Circles Forwards	20 reps
Arm Circles Backwards	20 reps
Thread the Needle	20 reps each way
Cervical Rotations 4-Pt or standing	20 reps
Arm Raises with Shoulder Blade Squeeze	20 reps

Mobility Routine: Lower Body

Body Weight Squats	20 reps
High Knees	20 reps
Half Kneeling Lunges Forward	20 reps each side
Knee to Wall Ankle Mobility	20 reps each side
Heel to Toe swipes (Hamstring)	20 reps each side

Stretching Routine: Upper Body

Arm Across Body	60 seconds each side
Arm Overhead	60 seconds each side
Pec Stretch	60 seconds
Child's Pose	60 seconds
Sleeper Stretch (For Shoulder	60 seconds each side

Stretching Routine: Lower Body

Quad Stretch	60 seconds each side
Hamstring Stretch	60 seconds each side
Groin Stretch	60 seconds each side
Glute Stretch (Figure Four)	60 seconds each side
Calf Stretch on Wall	60 seconds each side

Conclusion

Congratulations! If you have made is this far you have likely completed the whole program, where I can now say you went from couch to FIT!! As I alluded to in the week 8 coaching tips, this is just the beginning.

It is important to keep repeating week 8, while progressing the weights until you find a new program, such as my Fit to Barbell Basics – Building Power or another one that fits your needs.

The benefits of Strength Exercise are immense and should not be ignored.

If you have any questions about this program or how to progress you can reach out to me on all social media platforms @physiobrake

Exercise Descriptions

Dumbbell (DB) Bent Over Row

Start: Opposite hand and leg supported on bench. Neutral Spine.

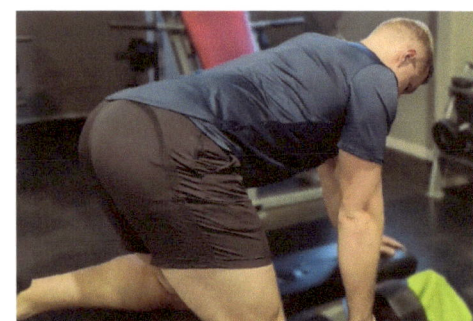

Movement: Pull the DB up to your body, keeping your elbow tucked.

Finish: Elbow bent 90 degrees with neutral wrist.

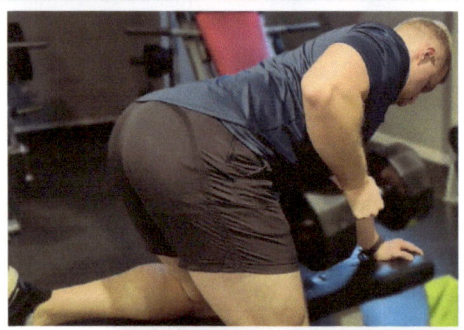

Kettle Bell (KB) Deadlift

Start: Standing tall, neutral spine, KB held with both hands, legs shoulder width apart.

Movement: Bend forward (hinging at the hips) by sticking your buttocks back as if you're trying to close the door with it.

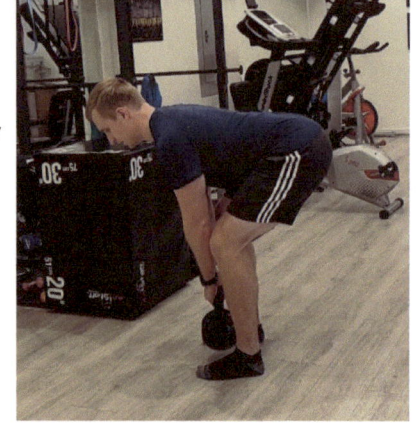

Finish: Small knee bend, neutral spine with your buttocks back, KB is centered between your legs.

DB Chest Press

Start: Arms straight pointed towards the ceiling. Core engaged, feet flat, and shoulder blades secure on the bench.

Movement: Lower the weight down with Elbows away from your body between A 45 to 75-degree angle

Finish: The elbows are just below your Trunk with the DB in line just above your chest.

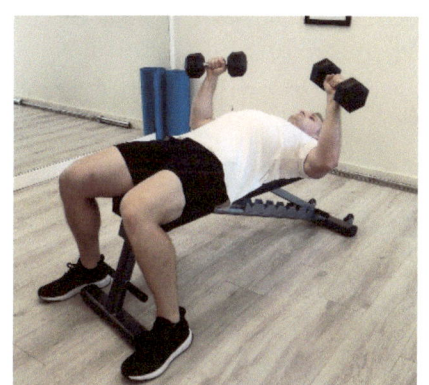

DB Shoulder Press

Start: Elbows 90 degrees from trunk and elbows bent 90 degrees. core engaged, small inward twist of the wrist so the DB Are on a slight angle

Movement: Press the weight straight up Overhead.

Finish: Finishing with elbows Straight, DB in the same plane as your body center. DB should not go behind your head.

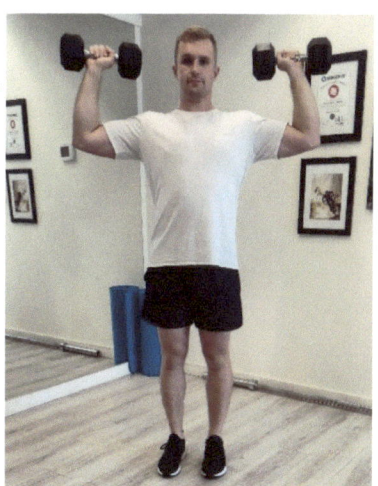

Cable (CB) Shoulder Rotation

Start: Elbow bent 90 degrees, elbow away from body at 90 degrees out to the side and cable (or band) is anchored low, down in front

Movement: Rotating your arm, thinking like the arm is on a spit, bring your fist pointing towards the ceiling. Try to avoid bending the wrist, keep them neutral

Finish: Elbow and armpit are square with a 90-degree angle. Wrist is neutral pointing toward the ceiling.

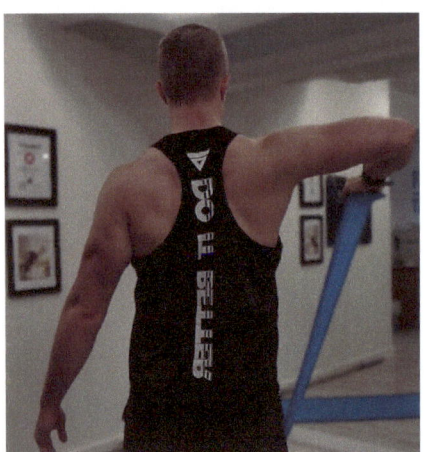 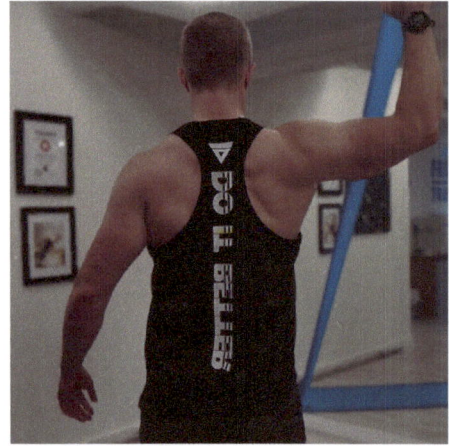

DB Squat

Start: Standing tall with DB's at your side and legs are shoulder width.

Movement: Squat by sticking your buttocks back like sitting into a chair.

Finish: Knee's straight, DB's at side, and spine neutral, but it is allowed to hinge forward.

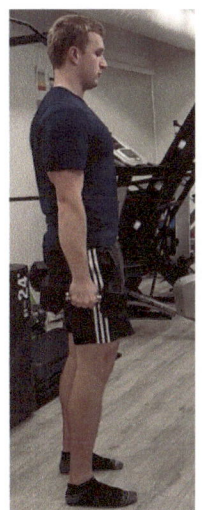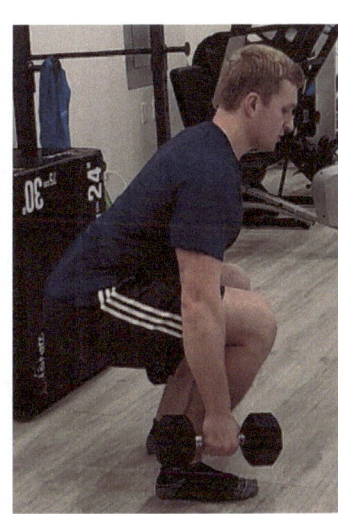

Reverse Lunge

Start: Standing tall with legs shoulder width apart.

Movement: Step back with the NON-working leg, this leg is providing balance only. Then push-off with the front leg by pushing down into the floor to engage the glutes and quads. Watch that your knee's stay pointing straight.

Finish: Back knee hovering off ground at 90 degrees'

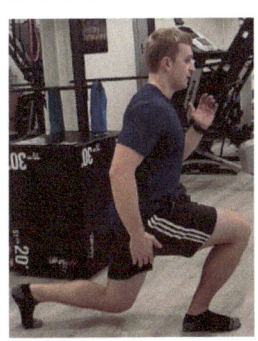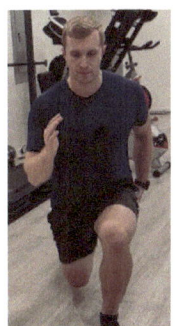

Dead Bug

Start: On your back with a neutral spine. Arms and legs pointing to the ceiling. Legs have a 90degree bend.

Movement: Extend opposite arm and leg straight out. Keeping your core engaged

Finish: Opposite arm and leg are pointing out, while the other remain in towards the ceiling.

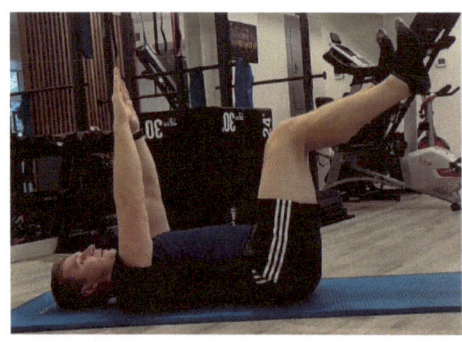

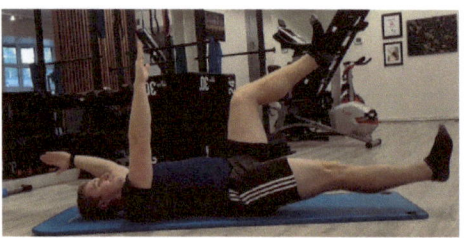

Heel Raises

Start: With one leg on the Edge of the step on tip toes. Knee straight.

Movement: Drop down so your heel goes below the height of the step.

Finish: Knee straight, heel is below the height of your step. You should feel the stretch in your calf.

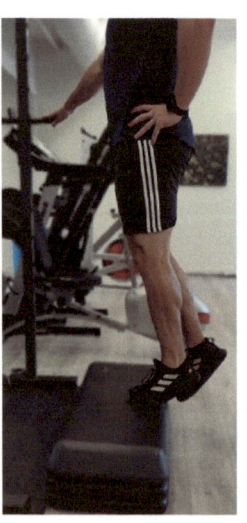 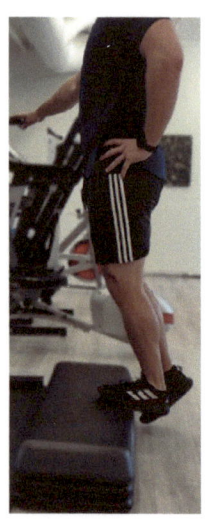

High Plank

Start, Finish, Movement:

Set your self up into push-up position With your spine neutral, shoulders square and hold this position.

Keep your core engaged throughout.

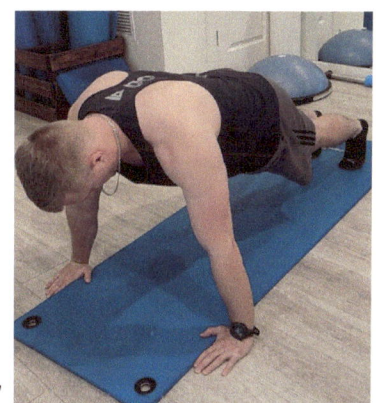

Lateral Lunge:

Start: Standing tall with your legs over shoulder width apart

Movement: Step to one side, sticking your buttocks back like you're sitting in a chair

Finish: You should be centered over one leg, buttocks back in a hinge position, neutral spine and toes are pointing forward.

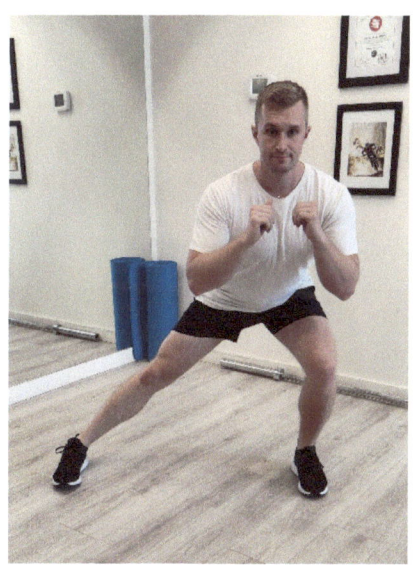

DB Pec Fly

Start: Laying on a bench with your spine neutral and arms pointing to the ceiling with wrist neutral

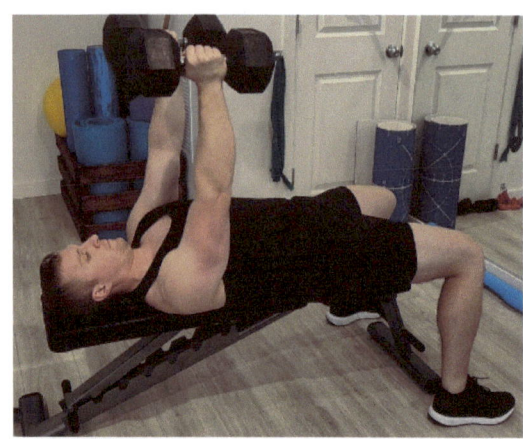

Movement: Bring the DB's down towards your side at an angle 45 to 75 degrees from your body keeping your wrist neutral and elbows going a little bit below the depth of your chest.

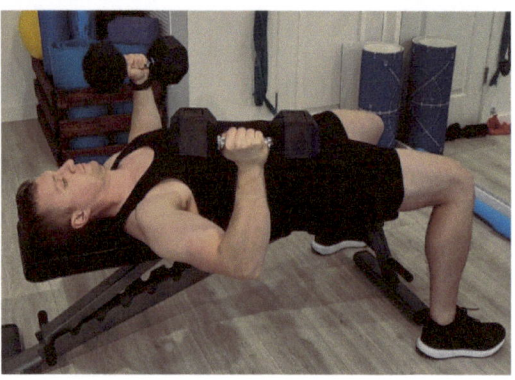

Finish: Elbow at bent 90 degrees, your elbows are also 45 to 75 degrees out from your body, slightly below the depth of your chest and core is engaged

Disclaimer

This gym-based exercise program is designed to be used by individuals who:
- Have medical clearance by their physician or other health care members to exercise and
- Do not have any comorbidities or contraindications to exercise.
- Understand gym safety.

By following this program, you are agreeing you have met the above criteria and are using it at your own risk.

This is not to be redistributed without explicit written consent of

Christopher Brake & **Erik Ottosen.**

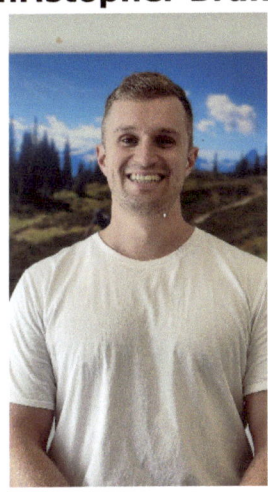
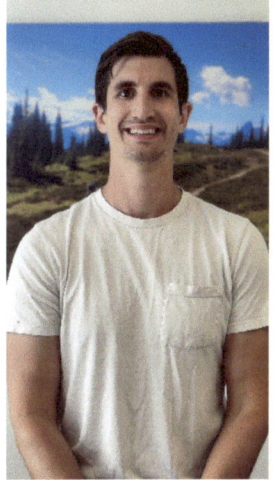

www.ingramcontent.com/pod-product-compliance
Lightning Source LLC
Chambersburg PA
CBHW040330220526
45473CB00009B/2636